Fish and Seafood
Keto Diet Cookbook

Delicious Low-Carbs, High Fat
Recipes for Your Ketogenic Diet

By Elisa Hayes

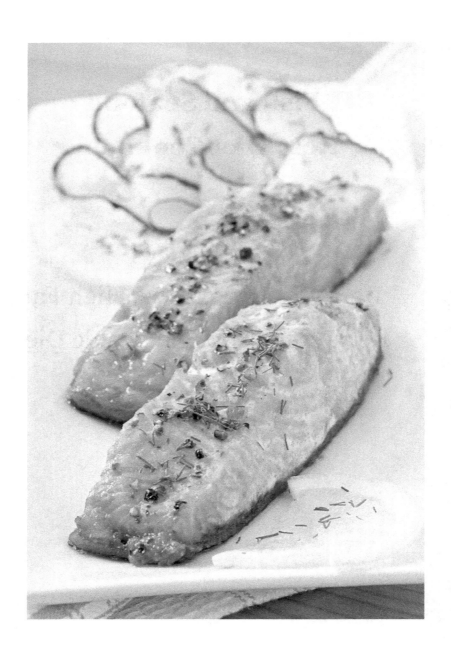

Table of Contents

The information in the following pages is broadly considered a truthful and accurate account of facts and as such, any inattention, use, or misuse of the information in question by the reader will render any resulting actions solely under their purview. There are no scenarios in which the publisher or the original author of this work can be in any fashion deemed liable for any hardship or damages that may befall them after undertaking information described herein.

Additionally, the information in the following pages is intended only for informational purposes and should thus be thought of as universal. As befitting its nature, it is presented without assurance regarding its prolonged validity or interim quality. Trademarks that are mentioned are done without written consent and can in no way be considered an endorsement from the trademark holder.

Introduction

The path to a perfect body and good physical health was very thorny for me. The only one wish which I was making for my birthdays for many years was to be a slim and beautiful girl. Alas, everything can't be as in fairy tales and the miracle didn't happen; my mirror was still showing the same fat, pimple girl. In childhood, the problem of being overweight didn't bother me much; I can say that I didn't care about it at all, I didn't know that weight would be momentous for me. I was an ordinary smiling child, playing with my peers, going to school, and traveling with my parents. That time my chubby cheeks seemed very sweet to everyone. But that was then. At 11-year-old, I went to middle school. New people, new teachers, I had no friends at all. Mentally I was broken. I counted the minutes until the end of the last lesson, to quickly sit in my mom's car and leave school. I started to eat a lot. Now I see that in this way I am stressed, but then the food serves as my antidepressant. Dozens of hamburgers, fried potatoes, coke – they were "my best friends". In addition to everything, I started to have horrible skin problems, it seemed to me that there was no place on my face wherever they hadn't appeared yet. Time passed and I no longer loved my reflection in the mirror even in 1%. I couldn't wear the clothes that I liked. I usually wore oversized shorts and t-shirts. I couldn't afford to wear a short dress and high heels. At 15-year-old I weighed more than 270lbs. I remember what I felt in those days, as it is happening now. I felt anger, irritation, hatred, and self-loathing. That prom party was the most terrible day of my life. Thank God it's over!

In those years, the keto diet was not very popular, fasting and drinking diets (which, as you already know, did not help me much) were more popular. Perhaps I wouldn't do anything, but my health problems were becoming more serious. It seemed that my body was simply screaming: please help me!

I remember the day that changed my life on a dime. I came to the clinic with pain in my stomach. But this time, I not only received painkillers but also found a mentor and friend. This was my physician. She had examined me and recommended that I go on a diet. I didn't want to do something and was categorically against it. However, my mind changed when she said: love your body, care about it, and it will thank you. What was my surprise when the diet turned out to be very simple to follow. Is it so easy to love myself? As you could understand I am talking about my favorite keto diet. Every day I was eating a maximum of proteins and a minimum of carbohydrates. That meant to consume meat, poultry, and fish and make restrictions for vegetables, fruits, and sweets. After 2 weeks, I lost 83lbs, and further results were getting better and better. All this time I was under the supervision of a doctor and this yielded results. A year later, I completely changed all the clothes in my wardrobe and oh my God I was able to wear a short dress and skirts! Now I can say that I am the happiest person. It happened because I fell in love with myself and started treating my body as a diamond. My life was filled with bright colors, I have a beloved husband, children, work, friends, I am healthy and like myself in the mirror. I am telling this story to prove that the right diet can solve almost all problems with body and health. It is a fact that our body is capable of dealing with dramatic changes, it is only worth loving. Never rest on your laurels, never give up and forbid people to say that you cannot do something. You are already a great fellow that you bought this cookbook and decided to take a step ahead in the direction to your dream. Let this book become your ray of hope, a lifesaver on the way to your wonderful transformation. If you believe in yourself and love your body, believe me, the result won't be long in coming. You will see in the mirror a completely new version of yourself, updated physically and mentally! Just trust the keto diet and your inner voice. Set a goal today and start the way of achieving it right now. Don't try to do it all in one time; let it be a small step day by day. Exactly now, this is the right time to start creating a new version of you. If this diet was able to change my life, I'm sure it will help you too!

Tuna Pie

Prep time: 10 minutes

Cook time: 30 minutes

Servings: 6

Ingredients:

- 3 spring onions, chopped
- 1 cup coconut flour
- ¼ cup of coconut oil
- 1 egg, beaten
- 1 teaspoon baking powder
- 9 oz tuna, canned, shredded

Method:

1. In the mixing bowl mix baking powder with coconut oil, and coconut flour. Knead the dough and put it in the non-stick baking pan. Flatten the dough in the shape of the pie crust.

2. Then mix shredded tuna with chopped spring onion and egg.

3. Put the fish mixture over the pie crust and flatten well.

4. Bake the pie at 360F for 30 minutes.

Nutritional info per serve: Calories 186, Fat 13.6, Fiber 1.2, Carbs 3.8, Protein 12.7

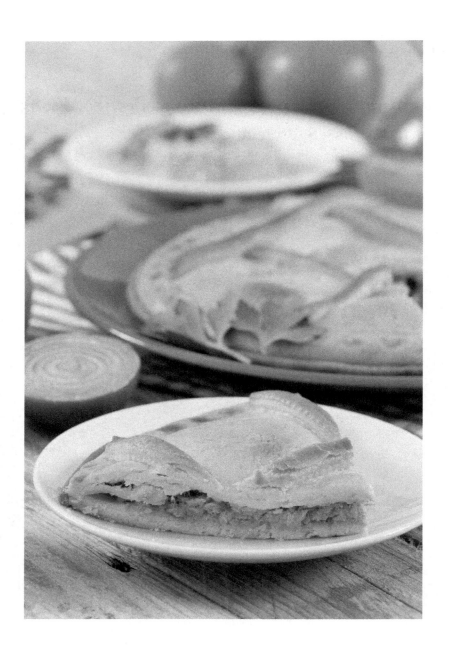

Wrapped Scallops

Prep time: 10 minutes

Cook time: 6 minutes

Servings: 4

Ingredients:

- 1-pound scallops
- 5 oz bacon, sliced
- 1 teaspoon ground coriander
- ½ teaspoon avocado oil

Method:

1. Sprinkle the scallops with ground coriander and wrap in the bacon. Secure scallops with the help of the toothpicks if needed.

2. Preheat the avocado oil well and put the scallops in it.

3. Roast them for 3 minutes per side.

Nutritional info per serve: Calories 292, Fat 15.7, Fiber 0, Carbs 3.2, Protein 32.2

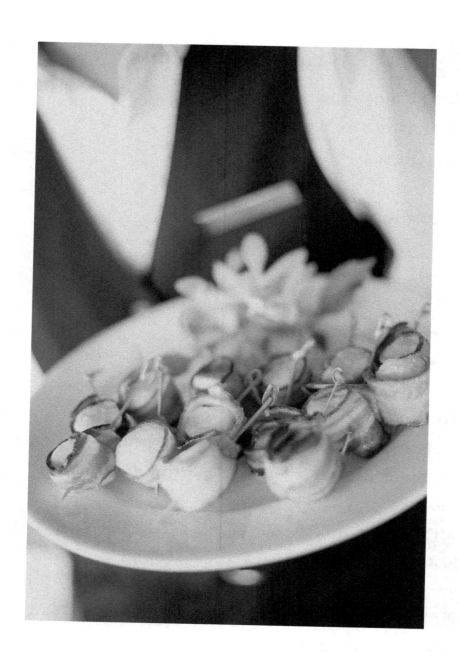

Lime Haddock

Prep time: 10 minutes

Cook time: 25 minutes

Servings: 4

Ingredients:

- 1-pound haddock
- 1 tablespoon avocado oil
- 1 teaspoon ground black pepper
- ½ teaspoon salt
- 1 lime

Method:

1. Sprinkle the haddock with avocado oil, ground black pepper, and salt and put in the lined with a baking paper baking tray.

2. Cut the lime into halves and squeeze over the fish.

3. Then sprinkle the fish with avocado oil and bake in the preheated 360F oven for 25 minutes.

Nutritional info per serve: Calories 138, Fat 1.5, Fiber 0.8, Carbs 2.3, Protein 27.7

Salmon Boats

Prep time: 10 minutes

Servings: 6

Ingredients:

- 6 celery stalks
- 8 oz salmon, canned
- 1 teaspoon scallions, chopped
- 1 tablespoon ricotta cheese

Method:

1. Shred the salmon and mix it with scallions and ricotta cheese.
2. Then fill the celery with salmon mixture.

Nutritional info per serve: Calories 56, Fat 2.6, Fiber 0.3, Carbs 0.7, Protein 7.8

Cheddar Tilapia

Prep time: 10 minutes

Cook time: 30 minutes

Servings: 4

Ingredients:

- 4 tilapia fillets, boneless
- ½ cup Cheddar cheese, shredded
- 1 teaspoon lemon juice
- 1 teaspoon dried thyme
- 1 teaspoon salt

Method:

1. Rub the tilapia fillets with dried thyme and salt.

2. Put them in the casserole mold.

3. After this, sprinkle the fish with lemon juice and shredded cheese. 4. Bake the tilapia for 30 minutes at 355F.

Nutritional info per serve: Calories 151, Fat 5.7, Fiber 0.1, Carbs 0.4, Protein 24.6

Salmon Kebabs

Prep time: 15 minutes

Cook time: 5 minutes

Servings:4

Ingredients:

- 1-pound salmon fillet
- 1 tablespoon marinara sauce
- 1 teaspoon avocado oil
- ¼ teaspoon ground cumin

Method:

1. Cut the salmon fillet into the medium cubes and mix with marinara sauce, avocado oil, and ground cumin.

2. String the fish cubes in the skewers and grill at 400F for 2 minutes per side.

Nutritional info per serve: Calories 155, Fat 7.3, Fiber 0.2,Carbs0.7,Protein22.1

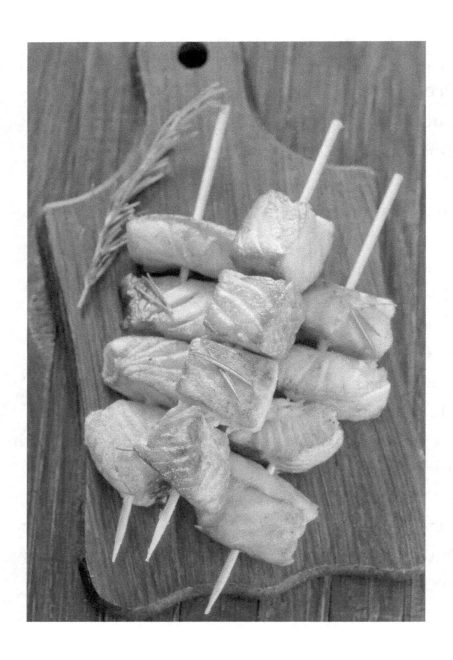

Soft Trout

Prep time: 10 minutes

Cook time: 25 minutes

Servings: 1

Ingredients:

- 3 oz trout fillet
- 2 tablespoons coconut oil
- ¼ cup coconut cream
- 1 teaspoon ground black pepper

Method:

1. Sprinkle the trout fillet with coconut oil, coconut cream, and ground black pepper.

2. Then put the fish and remaining mixture in the skillet and bake at 360F for 25 minutes.

Nutritional info per serve: Calories 539, Fat 48.8, Fiber 1.9, Carbs 4.7, Protein 24.3

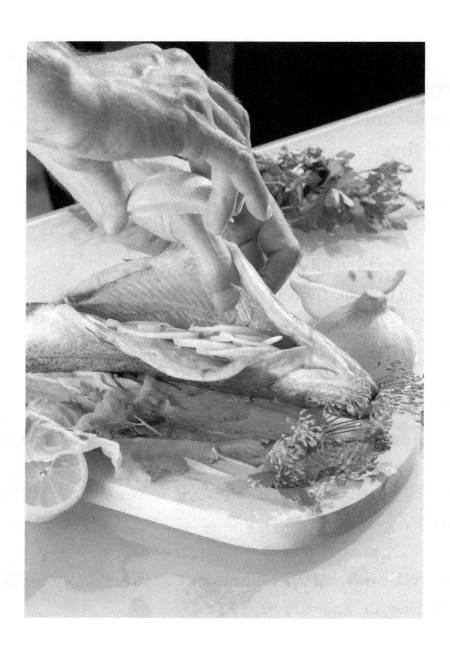

Cod in Sauce

Prep time: 5 minutes

Cook time: 20 minutes

Servings:2

Ingredients:

- 1-pound cod fillet
- 1 teaspoon keto tomato paste
- ½ cup coconut cream
- 1 teaspoon curry paste

Method:

1. Mix coconut cream with curry paste, and keto tomato paste and bring to boil.

2. Add cod and simmer the fish on medium heat for 15 minutes.

Nutritional info per serve: Calories 339, Fat 17.8, Fiber 1.4, Carbs 4.5, Protein 42.1

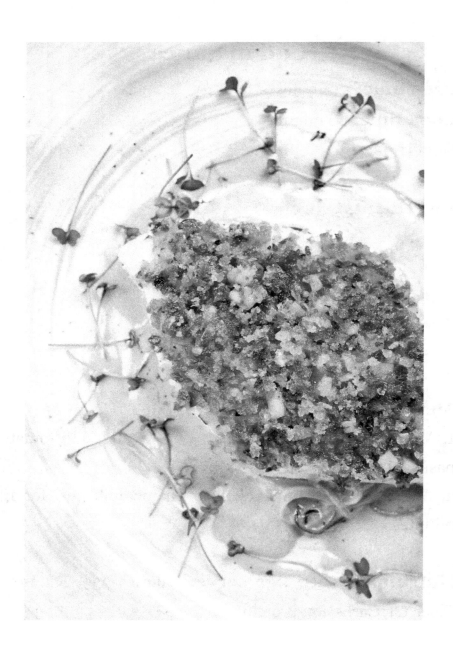

Lime Trout

Prep time: 10 minutes

Cook time: 30 minutes

Servings: 4

Ingredients:

- 4 trout fillets
- 1 lime
- 1 teaspoon dried thyme
- 1 teaspoon avocado oil

Method:

1. Slice the lime.

2. Put the trout fillets in the baking pan in one layer and sprinkle with avocado oil and dried thyme.

3. Then top it with sliced lime and bake at 360F for 30 minutes.

Nutritional info per serve: Calories 125, Fat 5.5, Fiber 0.6, Carbs 2, Protein 16.7

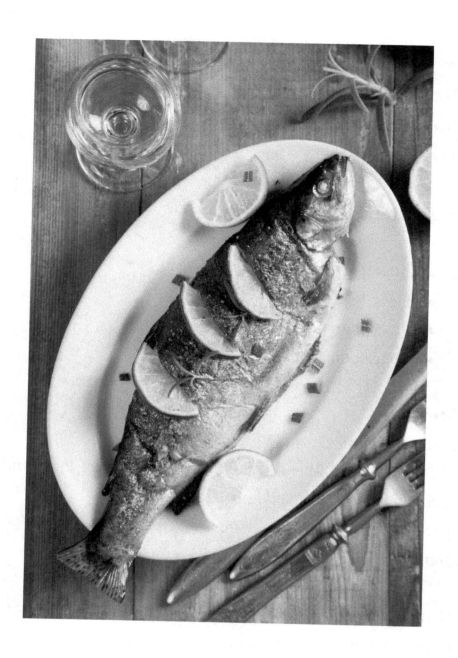

Cod with Chives

Prep time: 10 minutes

Cook time: 25 minutes

Servings:4

Ingredients:

- 4 cod fillets
- ½ lemon
- 1 rosemary, fresh
- 1 oz chives, chopped
- ½ cup coconut cream
- ½ teaspoon salt

Method:

1. Rub the cod fillets with rosemary, chives, and salt, and transfer in the baking pan.

2. Squeeze the lemon over the fish and add all remaining ingredients.

3. Cook the cod in the oven at 360F for 25 minutes.

Nutritional info per serve: Calories 164, Fat 8.3, Fiber 1.2, Carbs 2.8, Protein 21

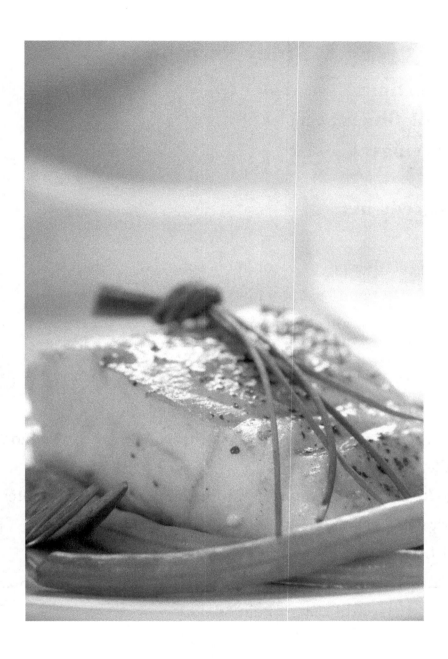

Spicy Salmon

Prep time: 10 minutes

Cook time: 12 minutes

Servings: 4

Ingredients:

- 2 tablespoons coconut oil, softened
- 1¼ pound salmon fillet
- 1 teaspoon chili powder

Method:

1. Sprinkle the salmon fillet with chili powder.

2. Then melt the coconut oil in the skillet and add salmon fillet.

3. Roast the salmon over the medium heat for 5 minutes per side.

Nutritional info per serve: Calories 473, Fat 26.2, Fiber 0.2, Carbs 0.4, Protein 60.6

Tilapia Bowl

Prep time: 10 minutes

Cook time: 10 minutes

Servings: 4

Ingredients:

- 9 oz tilapia fillet, chopped
- ½ cup white cabbage, shredded
- 1 teaspoon coconut oil
- 1 teaspoon chili powder
- ½ teaspoon cayenne pepper
- 1 cup coconut cream

Method:

1. Melt the coconut oil in the skillet.

2. Add tilapia and chili powder. Roast the fish for 2 minutes per side.

3. Then add cayenne pepper and cook the fish for 1 minute more.

4. Transfer the cooked tilapia in the bowl.

5. Add shredded cabbage and coconut cream.

6. Carefully mix the meal.

Nutritional info per serve: Calories 205, Fat 16.2, Fiber 1.8, Carbs 4.3, Protein 13.5

Salmon Meatballs

Prep time: 10 minutes

Cook time: 10 minutes

Servings: 4

Ingredients:

- 10 oz salmon, minced
- 1 teaspoon minced garlic
- 2 tablespoons coconut flour
- ½ teaspoon dried oregano
- ½ teaspoon dried cilantro
- 1 tablespoon coconut oil

Method:

1. In the mixing bowl, mix minced salmon, minced garlic, coconut flour, dried oregano, and cilantro.

2. Make the fish balls from the mixture.

3. Then preheat the coconut oil in the skillet well.

4. Add fish meatballs and roast them for 4 minutes per side over the low heat.

Nutritional info per serve: Calories 140, Fat 8.2, Fiber 1.6, Carbs 2.9, Protein 14.3

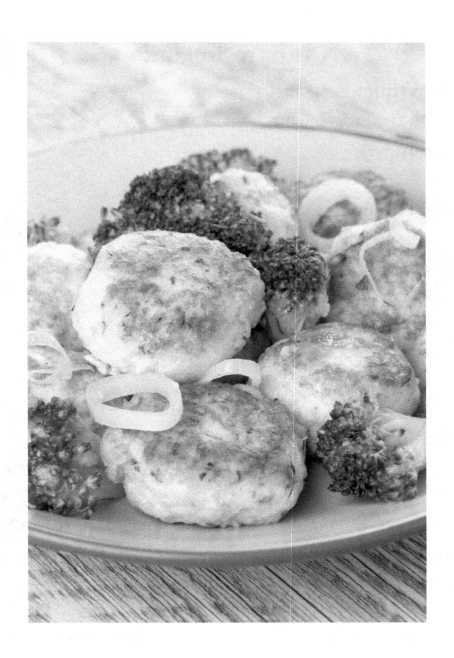

Cinnamon Hake

Prep time: 10 minutes

Cook time: 30 minutes

Servings:4

Ingredients:

- 4 hake fillets
- 1 teaspoon salt
- ½ teaspoon ground cinnamon
- 1 tablespoon coconut oil, melted
- ½ teaspoon chili powder

Method:

1. Brush the baking pan with coconut oil and put the hake fillets inside one layer.

2. Sprinkle the fish with salt, ground cinnamon, and chili powder.

3. Bake the fish at 360F for 30 minutes.

Nutritional info per serve: Calories 145, Fat 4.7, Fiber 0.3, Carbs 1.7, Protein 25.5

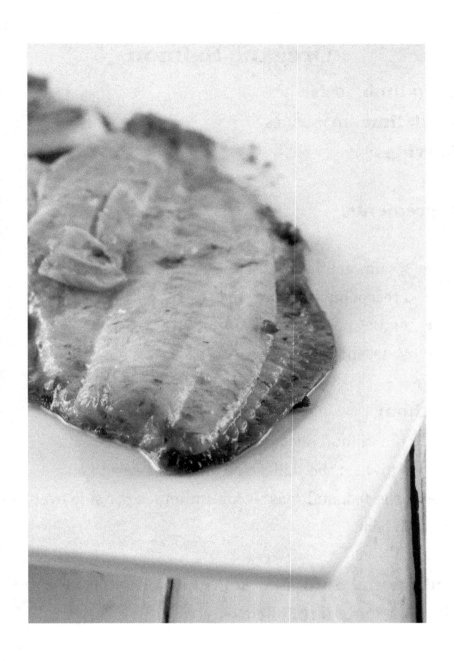

Oregano Salmon

Prep time: 10 minutes

Cook time: 10 minutes

Servings: 3

Ingredients:

- 3 salmon fillets
- 1 teaspoon dried oregano
- 1 tablespoon avocado oil
- ½ teaspoon salt

Method:

1. Rub the salmon fillets with dried oregano and salt.

2. Then preheat the skillet well and add avocado oil.

3. Add the fish and roast it for 4 minutes per side over the medium heat.

Nutritional info per serve: Calories 243, Fat 11.6, Fiber 0.4, Carbs 0.6, Protein 34.7

Sage Cod Fillets

Prep time: 10 minutes

Cook time: 30 minutes

Servings: 2

Ingredients:

- 2 cod fillets
- 1 teaspoon dried sage
- 1 tablespoon coconut aminos
- 1 tablespoon avocado oil

Method:

1. Mix dried sage with coconut aminos and avocado oil.

2. Then mix fish with coconut aminos mixture and leave for 10 minutes to marinate.

3. Bake the cod at 360F for 30 minutes.

Nutritional info per serve: Calories 108, Fat 1.9, Fiber 0.4, Carbs 2.1, Protein 20.1

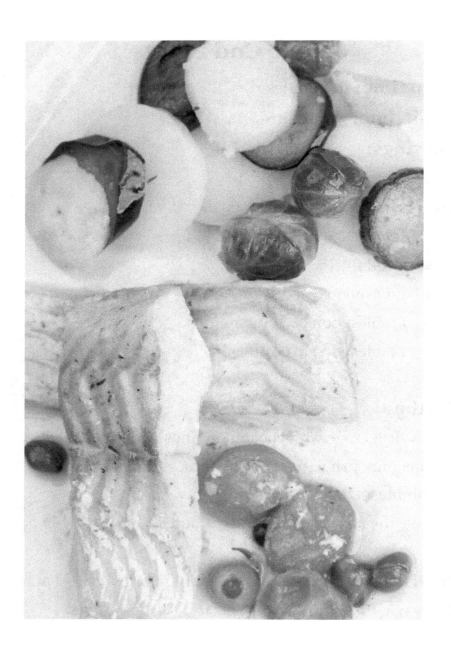

Herbed Oysters

Prep time: 5 minutes

Cook time: 10 minutes

Servings: 3

Ingredients:

- 6 oysters, shucked
- 1 teaspoon Italian seasonings
- 1 tablespoon dried cilantro
- 1 tablespoon coconut oil

Method:

1. Melt the coconut oil in the skillet and add oysters.

2. Sprinkle them with Italian seasonings and dried cilantro and roast for 7 minutes on medium heat. Stir them from time to time.

Nutritional info per serve: Calories 130, Fat 7.9, Fiber 0, Carbs 4.7, Protein 9.6

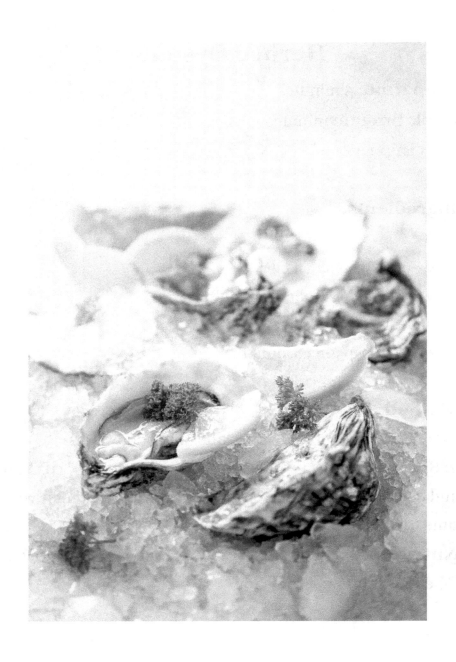

Cod Curry

Prep time: 10 minutes

Cook time: 25 minutes

Servings: 6

Ingredients:

- 1-pound cod fillet, chopped
- 1 tablespoon curry paste
- ½ teaspoon dried cilantro
- 1 teaspoon chili powder
- ½ bell pepper, diced
- 1 teaspoon coconut oil
- ½ cup coconut cream
- ½ teaspoon keto tomato paste

Method:

1. In the mixing bowl, mix keto tomato paste with coconut cream, chili powder, dried cilantro, and curry paste.

2. Then add cod and carefully mix the mixture. Add bell pepper and mix the mixture again.

3. Transfer it in the baking pan and bake at 360F for 25 minutes.

Nutritional info per serve: Calories 135, Fat 7.8, Fiber 0.7, Carbs 2.9, Protein 14.3

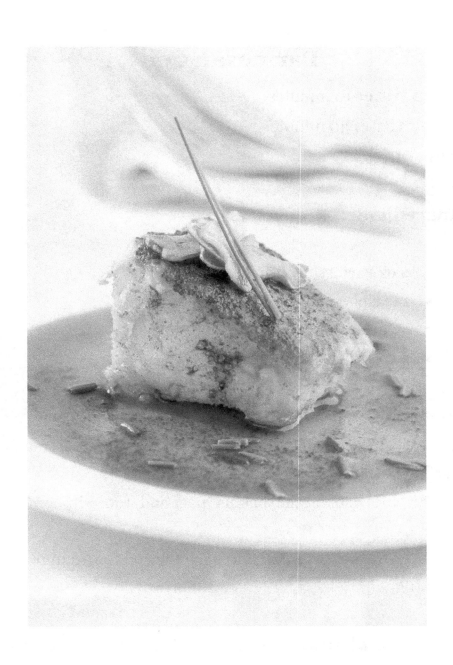

Parmesan Cod

Prep time: 10 minutes

Cook time: 30 minutes

Servings: 4

Ingredients:

- 2 oz Parmesan cheese, grated
- 1 teaspoon olive oil
- ½ teaspoon cayenne pepper
- 4 cod fillets

Method:

1. Brush the cod fillets with olive oil from each side and sprinkle with cayenne pepper.

2. Put the fish in the baking pan and top with grated cheese.

3. Cover the pan with foil and bake the cod for 30 minutes at 360F.

Nutritional info per serve: Calories 146, Fat 5.3, Fiber 0.1, Carbs 0.6, Protein 24.6

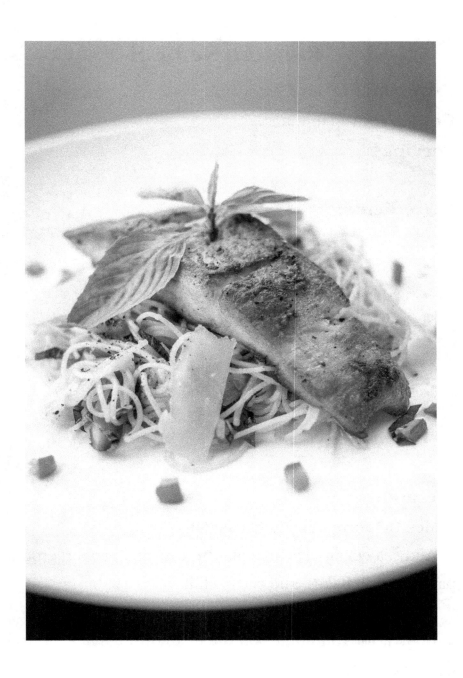

Roasted Sea Eel

Prep time: 10 minutes

Cook time: 15 minutes

Servings: 4

Ingredients:

- 10 oz sea eel
- 1 teaspoon cayenne pepper
- ½ teaspoon ground paprika
- ½ teaspoon chili flakes
- ½ teaspoon keto tomato paste
- 2 oz celery stalk, chopped
- 1 teaspoon coconut oil

Method:

1. Melt the coconut oil in the skillet.

2. Add sea eel and sprinkle it with cayenne pepper, ground paprika, chili flakes, and celery stalk.

3. Add keto tomato paste and carefully mix the mixture.

4. Cook it for 10 minutes on the medium-high heat or until the sea eel is tender.

Nutritional info per serve: Calories 182, Fat 11.9, Fiber 0.5, Carbs 1, Protein 17

Cilantro Salmon

Prep time: 10 minutes

Cook time: 8 minutes

Servings: 4

Ingredients:

- ½ teaspoon garlic powder
- 1-pound salmon fillet
- 1 tablespoon avocado oil
- 1 tablespoon dried cilantro

Method:

1. Sprinkle the salmon fillet with avocado oil, dried cilantro, and garlic powder.

2. Roast the fish in the well-preheat skillet for 4 minutes per side.

Nutritional info per serve: Calories 156, Fat 7.4, Fiber 0.2, Carbs 0.5, Protein 22.1

Italian Spices Seabass

Prep time: 10 minutes

Cook time: 40 minutes

Servings: 4

Ingredients:

- 1-pound sea bass
- 2 tablespoons butter
- 1 tablespoon Italian seasonings

Method:

1. Rub the sea bass with butter and Italian seasonings. Wrap it in the foil and put it in the baking tray.

2. Bake the fish at 360F for 40 minutes.

Nutritional info per serve: Calories 119, Fat 8.3, Fiber 0, Carbs 1.9, Protein 0.1

Mustard Cod

Prep time: 10 minutes

Cook time: 10 minutes

Servings: 4

Ingredients:

- 4 cod fillets
- 1 tablespoon mustard
- 1 tablespoon coconut cream
- 1 teaspoon avocado oil

Method:

1. Mix mustard with coconut cream.

2. Then mix cod fillets with mustard mixture and leave for 10 minutes to marinate.

3. Preheat the skillet well and put the avocado oil inside.

4. Add cod fillets and roast them for 5 minutes per side over the medium-low heat.

Nutritional info per serve: Calories 113, Fat 2.9, Fiber 0.5, Carbs 1.3, Protein 20.8

Shrimp Chowder

Prep time: 10 minutes

Cook time: 15 minutes

Servings:5

Ingredients:

- 7 oz cod fillet, chopped
- 5 oz shrimps, peeled
- 1 oz pancetta, chopped
- 1 spring onion, diced
- ½ cup celery stalk
- ½ cup heavy cream
- 3 cups of water

Method:

1. Roast the pancetta in the saucepan for 2 minutes per side.

2. Then add all remaining ingredients and carefully mix.

3. Cook the chowder on medium-low heat for 10 minutes.

Nutritional info per serve: Calories 144, Fat 7.7, Fiber 0.4, Carbs 2.2, Protein 16.1

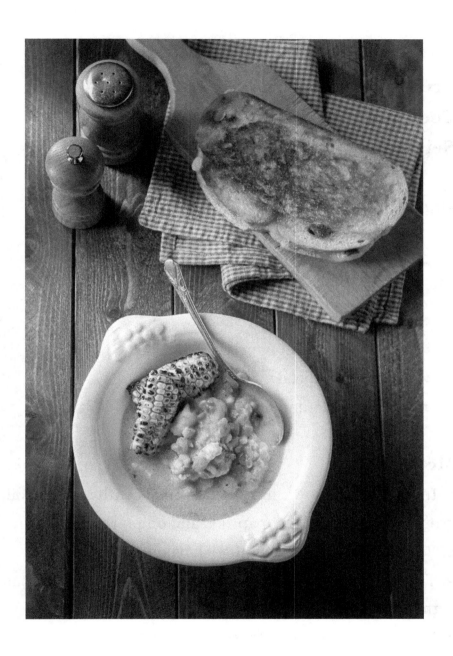

Onion Salmon

Prep time: 10 minutes

Cook time: 40 minutes

Servings: 4

Ingredients:

- 4 salmon fillets
- 1 tablespoon avocado oil
- 1 teaspoon ground coriander
- 1 teaspoon sweet paprika
- 2 scallions, diced
- 1 teaspoon onion powder

Method:

1. In the mixing bowl, mix salmon fillets with avocado oil, ground coriander, sweet paprika, and onion powder.
2. Put the mixture in the non-stick baking pan.
3. Then top the fish with scallions and cover the baking pan with foil.
4. Bake the salmon at 360F for 40 minutes.

Nutritional info per serve: Calories 249, Fat 11.5, Fiber 0.7, Carbs 2.3, Protein 34.9

Cheddar Pollock

Prep time: 10 minutes

Cook time: 25 minutes

Servings:3

Ingredients:

- 11 oz pollock fillet
- ½ cup Cheddar cheese, shredded
- 1 teaspoon white pepper
- 1 tablespoon avocado oil
- ¼ cup heavy cream

Method:

1. Brush the baking pan with avocado oil from inside.

2. Then slice the Pollock fillet and sprinkle it with white pepper.

3. Put the fish in the baking pan and top it with heavy cream and Cheddar cheese.

4. Cover the baking pan with foil and bake it at 360F for 25 minutes.

Nutritional info per serve: Calories 211, Fat 11.5, Fiber 0.4, Carbs 1.2, Protein 25.5

Parsley Tuna Fritters

Prep time: 10 minutes

Cook time: 10 minutes

Servings: 8

Ingredients:

- 12 ounces canned tuna, drained well and flaked
- 2 tablespoons fresh parsley, chopped
- 1 egg, beaten
- 2 tablespoons coconut oil
- 2 tablespoons coconut flour
- ½ teaspoon ground cumin

Method:

1. In the mixing bowl, mix canned tuna with parsley, egg, coconut flour, and cumin.

2. Then make the small fritters from the tuna mixture.

3. After this, melt the coconut oil in the skillet.

4. Add the tuna fritters and roast them for 4 minutes per side.

Nutritional info per serve: Calories 132, Fat 7.9, Fiber 1.3, Carbs 2.2, Protein 12.5

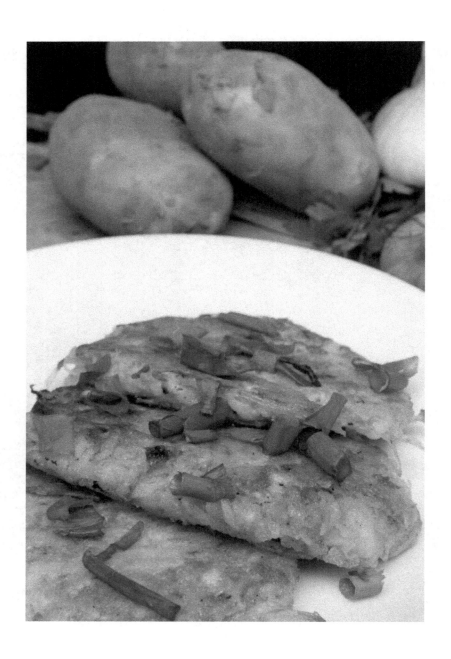

Clam Stew

Prep time: 5 minutes

Cook time: 15 minutes

Servings: 3

Ingredients:

- 5 oz clams
- ½ cup heavy cream
- ½ teaspoon curry paste
- ½ cup bell pepper, chopped
- 1 teaspoon keto tomato paste
- 1 cup of water
- 8 oz shrimps, peeled

Method:

1. Put all ingredients in the saucepan and bring to a boil.

2. Close the lid and simmer the stew for 5 minutes on the medium-low heat.

Nutritional info per serve: Calories 195, Fat 9.3, Fiber 0.5, Carbs 9, Protein 18.2

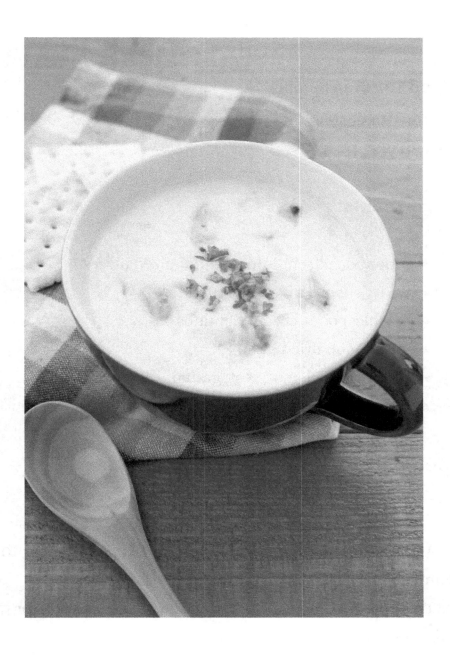

Sour Cod

Prep time: 15 minutes

Cook time: 10 minutes

Servings: 4

Ingredients:

- 1 pound cod, cut into medium-sized pieces
- ½ teaspoon chives, chopped
- 2 tablespoons coconut aminos
- 1 teaspoon dried dill
- ½ teaspoon lemon zest, grated
- 1 teaspoon avocado oil

Method:

1. Put the cod in the big bowl and sprinkle it with chives, coconut aminos, dried dill, and lemon zest.

2. Add avocado oil and carefully mix the fish. Leave it for 10 minutes to marinate.

3. Then preheat the skillet well, add fish and roast it for 5 minutes per side on medium heat.

Nutritional info per serve: Calories 129, Fat 1.1, Fiber 0.1, Carbs 1.8, Protein 26

Fennel Seabass

Prep time: 10 minutes

Cook time: 40 minutes

Servings:4

Ingredients:

- 1-pound sea bass
- 1 tablespoon fennel seeds
- 1 teaspoon avocado oil
- ½ teaspoon salt
- 1 teaspoon minced garlic

Method:

1. In the shallow bowl, mix fennel seeds with avocado oil, salt, and minced garlic.

2. Then carefully rub the seabass with fennel mixture and wrap in the foil.

3. Bake the seabass for 40 minutes at 360F.

Nutritional info per serve: Calories 65, Fat 1.9, Fiber 0.6, Carbs 2.6, Protein 0.3

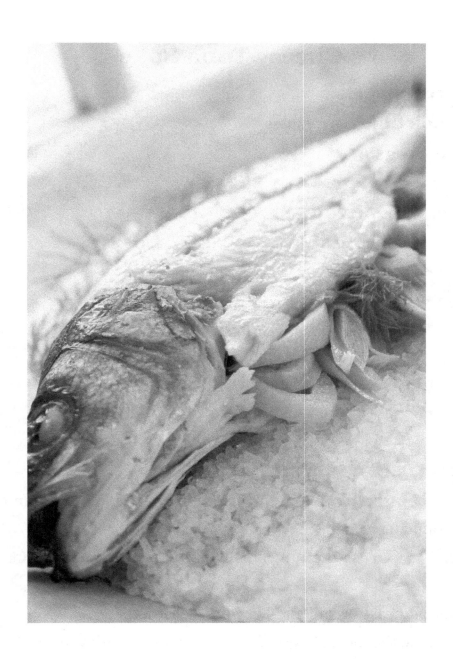

Cheesy Tuna Bake

Prep time: 10 minutes

Cook time: 25 minutes

Servings: 6

Ingredients:

- 4 oz Provolone cheese, grated
- 12 oz tuna fillet
- 1 teaspoon butter
- 1 teaspoon dried cilantro
- ½ teaspoon ground black pepper
- 1 tablespoon heavy cream

Method:

1. Chop the tuna and sprinkle it with dried cilantro and ground black pepper.

2. Then grease the ramekins with butter and put the tuna inside.

3. Add heavy cream and Provolone cheese.

4. Bake the meal at 360F for 25 minutes or until you get the crunchy crust.

Nutritional info per serve: Calories 287, Fat 24.2, Fiber 0.1, Carbs 0.6, Protein 16.8

Parsley Sea Bass

Prep time: 10 minutes

Cook time: 30 minutes

Servings: 4

Ingredients:

- ¼ lime, sliced
- 1-pound sea bass fillet
- 1 tablespoon dried parsley
- 1 teaspoon avocado oil
- ¼ teaspoon salt

Method:

1. Brush the sea bass fillet with avocado oil and put it in the casserole mold.

2. Top the fish with sliced lime and sprinkle with salt and dried parsley.

3. Bake the fish at 355F for 30 minutes.

Nutritional info per serve: Calories 144, Fat 3.1, Fiber 0.2, Carbs 0.6, Protein 26.9

Scallions Salmon Cakes

Prep time: 10 minutes

Cook time: 10 minutes

Servings:4

Ingredients:

- 8 oz salmon, canned, shredded
- 2 tablespoons almond flour
- 2 oz scallions, chopped
- 1 teaspoon ground coriander
- ½ teaspoon salt
- 1 egg, beaten
- 1 tablespoon coconut oil

Method:

1. In the mixing bowl, mix shredded salmon with almond flour, scallions, ground salt, and egg.

2. Then melt the coconut oil in the skillet well.

3. Make the small cakes from the salmon mixture with the help of the spoon and transfer them in the skillet.

4. Roast the salmon cakes for 3 minutes per side or until they are light brown.

Nutritional info per serve: Calories 205, Fat 15, Fiber 1.9, Carbs 4.1, Protein 15.6

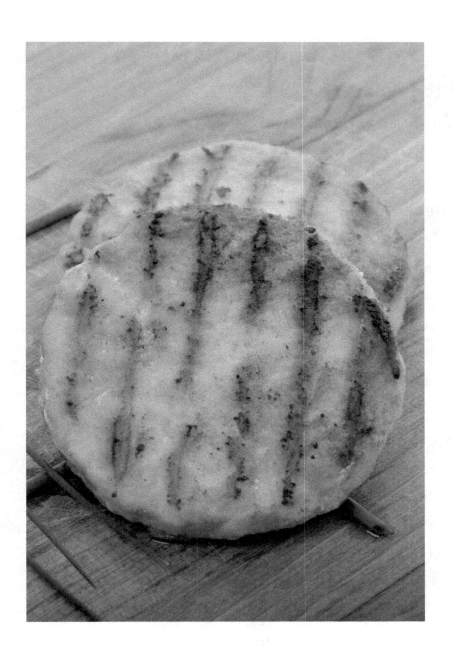

Tilapia with Olives

Prep time: 10 minutes

Cook time: 20 minutes

Servings: 2

Ingredients:

- 2 tilapia fillets
- 1 tablespoon avocado oil
- 2 kalamata olives, sliced
- 1 teaspoon apple cider vinegar
- 1 teaspoon ground turmeric

Method:

1. Rub the tilapia fillets with ground turmeric and sprinkle with apple cider vinegar.

2. Then brush the baking pan with avocado oil from inside and put the fish.

3. Top it with olives and bake at 360F for 20 minutes.

Nutritional info per serve: Calories 112, Fat 2.5, Fiber 0.7, Carbs 1.4, Protein 21.2

Cod Sticks

Prep time: 10 minutes

Cook time: 15 minutes

Servings:6

Ingredients:

- 10 oz cod fillet
- ½ cup almond flour
- 2 eggs, beaten
- 1 teaspoon salt
- ½ teaspoon smoked paprika
- 3 oz Parmesan, grated
- 1 teaspoon butter

Method:

1. Cut the cod fillet into the sticks and sprinkle with salt and smoked paprika.

2. Then dip the fish sticks in the eggs and coat in the almond flour and Parmesan.

3. Grease the baking tray with butter and put the fish sticks inside.

4. Bake the meal at 360F for 10-15 minutes or until the cod sticks are crunchy.

Nutritional info per serve: Calories 124, Fat 6.7, Fiber 0.3, Carbs 1.2, Protein 15.4

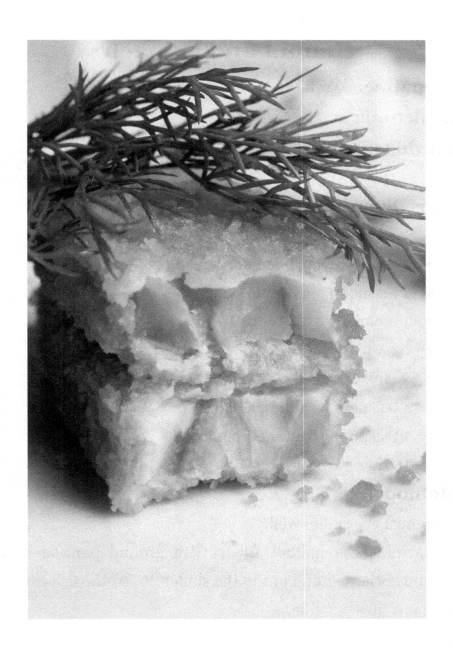

Halibut and Spinach

Prep time: 10 minutes

Cook time: 15 minutes

Servings: 2

Ingredients:

- 1 yellow bell pepper, seeded and chopped
- 1 teaspoon apple cider vinegar
- 1 tablespoon avocado oil
- 2 halibut fillets
- 2 cups spinach, chopped
- 1 teaspoon ground paprika
- 1 teaspoon ground coriander

Method:

1. Preheat the skillet well.

2. Sprinkle the halibut fillets with ground paprika and ground coriander and put in the skillet. Roast the fish fillets for 2 minutes per side.

3. Then add bell pepper, apple cider vinegar, and spinach.

4. Cover the skillet with foil and bake at 360F for 10 minutes.

Nutritional info per serve: Calories 357, Fat 8, Fiber 2.2, Carbs 6.6, Protein 62.2

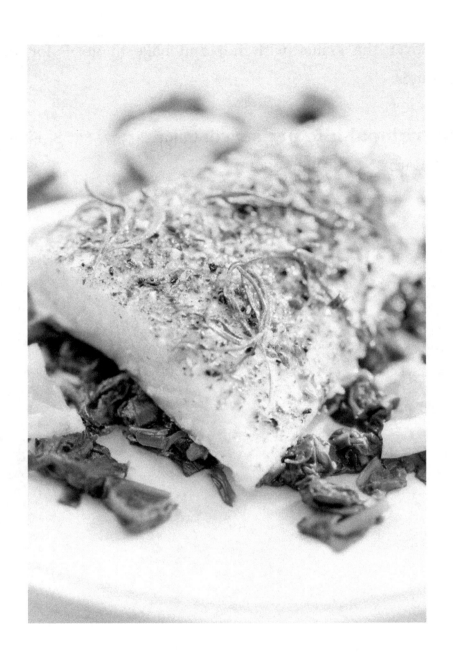

Coriander Cod

Prep time: 15 minutes

Cook time: 10 minutes

Servings: 2

Ingredients:

- 12 oz cod fillet
- 1 tablespoon coconut oil
- 1 tablespoon ground coriander
- 1 teaspoon dried dill
- 1 teaspoon coconut aminos

Method:

1. Sprinkle the cod fillet with ground coriander, dried dill, and coconut aminos.

2. Leave the fish for 10 minutes to marinate.

3. After this, melt the coconut oil in the skillet and add marinated fish.

4. Roast it for 5 minutes per side on the medium heat.

Nutritional info per serve: Calories 199, Fat 8.3, Fiber 0.1, Carbs 0.8, Protein 30.5

White Fish Stew

Prep time: 10 minutes

Cook time: 40 minutes

Servings: 4

Ingredients:

- 4 tilapia fillets
- ½ cup turnip, chopped
- 1 cup of water
- 1 teaspoon avocado oil
- 2 spring onions, diced
- 1 teaspoon ground black pepper
- ½ teaspoon salt
- 1 teaspoon keto tomato paste

Method:

1. Mix water with keto tomato paste in the saucepan.

2. Add fish, turnip, avocado oil, spring onion, ground black pepper, and salt.

3. Close the lid and cook the stew on low heat for 40 minutes.

Nutritional info per serve: Calories 113, Fat 1.3, Fiber 1.1, Carbs 4.3, Protein 21.6

Crab Fritters

Prep time: 10 minutes

Cook time: 12 minutes

Servings:4

Ingredients:

- 4 tablespoons ricotta cheese
- 1 teaspoon garlic powder
- 8 oz crab meat, canned, shredded
- 2 oz provolone cheese, shredded
- 1 teaspoon dried dill

Method:

1. Line the baking tray with baking paper.

2. Then mix ricotta cheese, garlic powder, shredded crab meat, provolone cheese, and dried dill.

3. Make the fritters from the mixture and put them in the baking tray.

4. Bake the crab fritters in the preheated to 360F oven for 12 minutes.

Nutritional info per serve: Calories 125, Fat 6, Fiber 0.1, Carbs 2.8, Protein 12.7

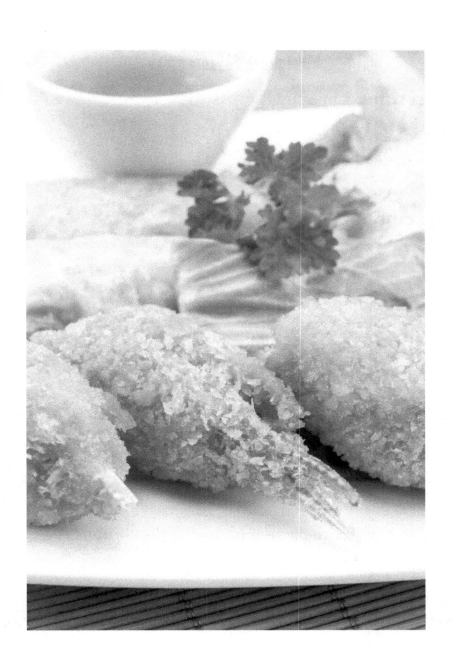

Lime Shrimp

Prep time: 5 minutes

Cook time: 10 minutes

Servings: 4

Ingredients:

- 1-pound shrimps, peeled
- ½ lemon
- 1 tablespoon butter
- ½ teaspoon chili powder

Method:

1. Melt the butter in the saucepan and add shrimps.

2. Sprinkle the shrimps with chili powder and roast for 2 minutes per side.

3. Then squeeze the lemon juice over the shrimps and cook them for 5 minutes more.

Nutritional info per serve: Calories 163, Fat 4.9, Fiber 0.3, Carbs 2.6, Protein 26

Ginger Cod

Prep time: 10 minutes

Cook time: 30 minutes

Servings: 4

Ingredients:

- 4 cod fillets
- 1 teaspoon minced ginger
- 2 tablespoons butter
- 1 teaspoon ground black pepper
- 1 teaspoon ground turmeric

Method:

1. In the shallow bowl, mix minced ginger, butter, ground black pepper, and ground turmeric.

2. Rub the cod fillets with the ginger mixture and wrap in the foil.

3. Bake the fish for 30 minutes at 360F.

Nutritional info per serve: Calories 146, Fat 6.9, Fiber 0.3, Carbs 1, Protein 20.2

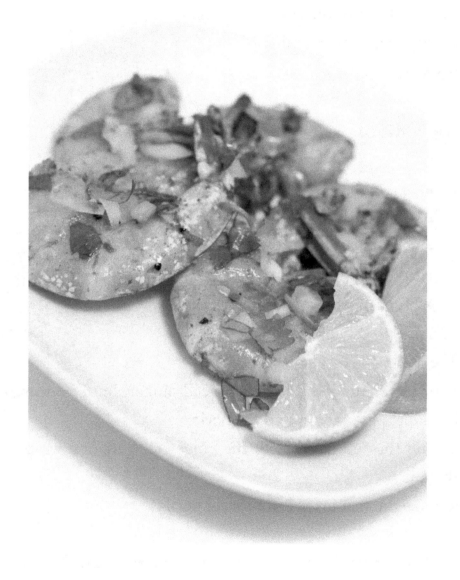

Tomato Sea Bass

Prep time: 10 minutes

Cook time: 35 minutes

Servings: 4

Ingredients:

- 2 sea bass fillets
- 1 tablespoon keto tomato paste
- 1 tablespoon butter, softened
- ½ teaspoon ground black pepper
- ½ teaspoon dried rosemary

Method:

1. Rub the sea bass fillets with ground black pepper and dried rosemary.

2. Then sprinkle the fish with butter and keto tomato paste. Wrap the sea bass in the foil.

3. Bake the fish at 360F for 35 minutes.

Nutritional info per serve: Calories 93, Fat 4.2, Fiber 0.3, Carbs 1, Protein 12.2

Scallions Salmon Spread

Prep time: 15 minutes

Cook time: 0 minutes

Servings:6

Ingredients:

- 1-pound salmon, canned, shredded
- 1 oz scallions, diced
- 1 tablespoon butter, softened
- 1 tablespoon ricotta cheese
- ½ teaspoon minced garlic
- ¼ teaspoon lime zest, grated

Method:

1. Put all ingredients in the food processor and blend until smooth.

2. Then transfer it in the bowl and refrigerate for 10-15 minutes before serving.

Nutritional info per serve: Calories 122, Fat 6.8, Fiber 0.1, Carbs 0.6, Protein 15.1

Tomato and Thyme Shrimps

Prep time: 10 minutes

Cook time: 10 minutes

Servings: 4

Ingredients:

- 1-pound shrimps
- 1 teaspoon dried thyme
- 1 teaspoon coconut oil
- 1 teaspoon keto tomato paste
- ¼ cup of coconut milk

Method:

1. Melt the coconut oil in the saucepan and add shrimps.

2. Then sprinkle them with dried thyme, keto tomato paste, and coconut milk.

3. Stir the mixture until you get tomato color.

4. Cook the shrimps on medium heat for 5 minutes.

Nutritional info per serve: Calories 181, Fat 6.7, Fiber 0.5, Carbs 3, Protein 26.3

Chili Cod

Prep time: 10 minutes

Cook time: 6 minutes

Servings:1

Ingredients:

- 1 cod fillet
- 1 teaspoon coconut oil, melted
- ½ teaspoon garlic powder
- ½ teaspoon chili powder
- ½ teaspoon coconut aminos

Method:

1. Rub the cod fillet with chili powder and garlic powder.

2. Then sprinkle it with coconut oil and coconut aminos.

3. Preheat the skillet well and put the fish inside.

4. Roast it for 3 minutes per side on high heat.

Nutritional info per serve: Calories 143, Fat 5.8, Fiber 0.6, Carbs 2.2, Protein 21.4

Shrimp Bowl

Prep time: 10 minutes

Cook time: 5 minutes

Servings: 4

Ingredients:

- ½ cup celery stalk, chopped
- 1 spring onion, sliced
- 1 tablespoon avocado oil
- 10 oz shrimps, peeled
- 1 teaspoon ground coriander
- 1 tablespoon coconut oil

Method:

1. Melt the coconut oil in the skillet.

2. Add shrimps and ground coriander. Roast the seafood for 5 minutes. Stir it from time to time.

3. Then transfer the shrimps in the bowl and add all remaining ingredients.

4. Carefully mix the meal.

Nutritional info per serve: Calories 123, Fat 5.1, Fiber 0.5, Carbs 2.3, Protein 16.4

Tender Catfish

Prep time: 10 minutes

Cook time: 10 minutes

Servings: 7

Ingredients:

- 1-pound catfish, chopped
- ½ cup coconut cream
- 1 teaspoon ground turmeric
- ½ teaspoon smoked paprika

Method:

1. Bring the coconut cream to boil.

2. Meanwhile, sprinkle the catfish with ground turmeric and smoked paprika.

3. Put the fish in the boiling coconut cream and cook for 10 minutes on medium heat.

Nutritional info per serve: Calories 189, Fat 12.8, Fiber 1, Carbs 6.4, Protein 12.2

Cayenne Mahi Mahi

Prep time: 10 minutes

Cook time: 8 minutes

Servings: 2

Ingredients:

- 2 mahi-mahi fillets
- 1 teaspoon cayenne pepper
- 1 tablespoon coconut oil
- 1 teaspoon salt

Method:

1. Melt the coconut oil in the skillet.

2. Then sprinkle the fish fillets with cayenne pepper and salt.

3. Roast the fish fillets in the hot coconut oil for 4 minutes per side.

Nutritional info per serve: Calories 150, Fat 7.9, Fiber 0.2, Carbs 0.5, Protein 19

Sweet Salmon Steaks

Prep time: 10 minutes

Cook time: 6 minutes

Servings:4

Ingredients:

- 4 salmon fillets (steaks)
- ½ teaspoon Erythritol
- 1 tablespoon water
- 1 teaspoon ground black pepper
- 1 teaspoon smoked paprika
- ¼ cup coconut cream
- 1 teaspoon coconut oil

Method:

1. In the mixing bowl, mix Erythritol, ground black pepper, and smoked paprika.

2. Rub the salmon fillets with mixture and then put in the skillet.

3. Add coconut oil and coconut cream.

4. Roast the fish for 5 minutes per side on the medium heat.

Nutritional info per serve: Calories 283, Fat 15.8, Fiber 0.7, Carbs 1.5, Protein 35

Pepper Shrimp

Prep time: 10 minutes

Cook time: 5 minutes

Servings: 2

Ingredients:

- ½ pound shrimp, peeled and deveined
- 1 tablespoon lime juice
- 1 teaspoon ground black pepper
- 2 tablespoons avocado oil

Method:

1. Preheat the skillet well and add avocado oil.

2. Add shrimps and sprinkle them with ground black pepper.

3. Roast the shrimps for 2 minutes per side.

4. Sprinkle the cooked shrimps with lime juice.

Nutritional info per serve: Calories 156, Fat 3.7, Fiber 0.9, Carbs 3.2, Protein 26.1

Jalapeno Tilapia

Prep time: 10 minutes

Cook time: 20 minutes

Servings:4

Ingredients:

- 2 jalapenos, chopped
- 1/3 avocado, pitted, sliced
- 1 tablespoon lime juice
- 4 tilapia fillets
- 1 tablespoon avocado oil

Method:

1. Brush the baking pan with avocado oil.

2. Then put the tilapia fillets inside.

3. Sprinkle them with lime juice and top with jalapeno peppers.

4. Bake the tilapia for 20 minutes at 360F.

5. Then top the cooked fish with avocado.

Nutritional info per serve: Calories 159, Fat 7.8, Fiber 1.3, Carbs 1.9, Protein 21.4